SWITCH ON
YOUR BRAIN
·WORKBOOK·

SWITCH ON YOUR BRAIN
• WORKBOOK •

The Key to Peak Happiness, Thinking, and Health

Dr. Caroline Leaf

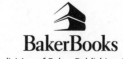

BakerBooks

a division of Baker Publishing Group
Grand Rapids, Michigan

Published by Baker Books
a division of Baker Publishing Group
PO Box 6287, Grand Rapids, MI 49516-6287
www.bakerbooks.com

Printed in the United States of America

Library of Congress Cataloging-in-Publication Data is on file at the Library of Congress, Washington, DC.

ISBN 978-0-8010-7547-6

Unless otherwise indicated, Scripture quotations are from the New King James Version®. Copyright © 1982 by Thomas Nelson, Inc. Used by permission. All rights reserved.

Scripture quotations labeled AMP are from the Amplified® Bible, copyright © 2015 by The Lockman Foundation. Used by permission. (www.Lockman.org)

Scripture quotations labeled ESV are from The Holy Bible, English Standard Version® (ESV®), copyright © 2001 by Crossway, a publishing ministry of Good News Publishers. Used by permission. All rights reserved. ESV Text Edition: 2011

Scripture quotations labeled MSG are from THE MESSAGE. Copyright © by Eugene H. Peterson 1993, 1994, 1995, 1996, 2000, 2001, 2002. Used by permission of NavPress. All rights reserved. Represented by Tyndale House Publishers, Inc.

Scripture quotations labeled NIV are from the Holy Bible, New International Version®. NIV®. Copyright © 1973, 1978, 1984, 2011 by Biblica, Inc.™ Used by permission of Zondervan. All rights reserved worldwide. www.zondervan.com

Scripture quotations labeled NLT are from the *Holy Bible*, New Living Translation, copyright © 1996, 2004, 2015 by Tyndale House Foundation. Used by permission of Tyndale House Publishers, Inc., Carol Stream, Illinois 60188. All rights reserved.

All emphasis in Scripture has been added by the author.

Portions of this text have been taken from *Switch On Your Brain*, published by Baker Books, 2013.

The information and solutions offered in this book are the result of years of research, practical application, and clinical work. The information in this book is intended to serve as guidelines for managing toxic thoughts, emotions, and bodies, and not as a replacement for professional medical advice or therapy. Please discuss specific symptoms and medical conditions with your doctor. Any use of this information is at the user's discretion. Switch On Your Brain LLC and the author make no representations or warranties that any individual will achieve a particular result. Any and all express or implied warranties, including the warranties of merchantability and fitness for a particular purpose, are disclaimed. Switch On Your Brain LLC and the author specifically disclaim any and all liability arising directly or indirectly from the use or application of any information contained in this book.

In keeping with biblical principles of creation stewardship, Baker Publishing Group advocates the responsible use of our natural resources. As a member of the Green Press Initiative, our company uses recycled paper when possible. The text paper of this book is composed in part of post-consumer waste.

20 21 22 23   7

Contents

Prologue   7

Introduction   9

KEY 1: Mind Controls Matter   17

KEY 2: Choice and Your Multiple-Perspective Advantage   25

KEY 3: Your Choices Change Your Brain   35

KEY 4: Catch Those Thoughts   45

KEY 5: Entering into Directed Rest   53

KEY 6: Stop Milkshake-Multitasking   61

KEY 7: Thinking, God, and the Quantum Physics Brain   69

KEY 8: The Science of Thought   81

The 21-Day Brain Detox   89

21-Day Detox Worksheet Example   103

Conclusion   107

Recommended Reading   109

Prologue

*W*hat would you do if you found a switch that could turn on your brain and enable you to be happier, healthier in your mind and body, more prosperous, and more intelligent? I began my book *Switch On Your Brain* with this simple yet profound question. Of course, we all want to be happier and healthier, but we often do not know how to go about bettering our lives. Millions of books, shows, magazines, and programs promise the key to happiness and success, yet they often fall short of producing true change. We feel great for a few days or weeks, but very soon the circumstances of life come crashing down on us and we once again feel crushed under their weight.

Yet we cannot change anything unless we change our thinking. In *Switch On Your Brain*, I describe how important our mind is for peak health and how our thoughts can impact every area of our lives. Regardless of what happens in our lives, we can *choose* how we react to our circumstances. "God has not given us a spirit of fear, but of power and of love and of a *sound mind*" (2 Tim. 1:7). We are more than conquerors in Him (Rom. 8:37). We can renew our minds through the help of the Holy Spirit and renew our world (Rom. 12:2). When we start to change our thinking, we can truly transform our lives.

I created this workbook as a guide to help you understand and apply the principles of renewed thinking in *Switch On Your Brain*. Each key follows the chapters in the book, with the science, linked Scripture context, and a series of questions that will help you understand and apply the principles of renewed thinking in the second part of the book, the 21-Day Brain Detox. Be as specific as you can as you answer the questions, because research shows change will happen when we dig deep to find the root of issues. Once you have completed these questions, there is a discussion section, which will draw on Scripture to help you see the connection between science and the Bible. I would recommend working through the questions and Scripture discussions a second time, after you have completed the workbook and as you use the 21-Day Brain Detox program, which will help you better understand and apply the principles in *Switch On Your Brain*.

I have used multiple translations of the Bible throughout this study guide. If you wish to use a different translation, translate the Scripture yourself, or use multiple versions of the same Scripture, you are more than welcome! Shifting between translations forces us to analyze Scripture from a variety of different viewpoints, which increases mind health.

At the end of the workbook, there is a recommended reading list for those who wish to dig deeper into the key points I have written about in *Switch On Your Brain* and this workbook. There are two sections: science/philosophy and theology/philosophy. Many of these sources can be found in the bibliography and notes in *Switch On Your Brain*, but I have highlighted the most important books and articles and added a few new sources I have researched since writing *Switch On Your Brain* in 2013.

Of course, the crucial principle to remember as you go through this workbook, as well as the book and the twenty-one-day program, is that change only occurs when we *want* to change. Although this may sound redundant, I have come across many people in my practice and my travels who like the idea of changing the way they think and transforming their lives but are not desperate enough to truly change. God has given us the incredible gift of free will, and it is up to us how we use it. We can *choose* life or death (Deut. 30:19).

No one can change your thinking—and your life—except *you*.

Introduction

See pages 19–28 in *Switch On Your Brain*.

Main Scripture: Faith is the substance of things *hoped* for, the evidence of things not seen. (Heb. 11:1)

Linked Science Concept: Thoughts are real, physical things that occupy mental real estate. Moment by moment, every day, you are changing the structure of your brain through your thinking. When we *hope*, it is an activity of the mind that changes the structure of our brain in a positive and normal direction.

1. *It was only a few decades ago that scientists considered the brain to be a fixed and hardwired machine. This view saw the damaged brain as incurable and the focus was compensation, not restoration of function.* How do these theories shape the way we view humanity? How does this way of thinking impact our view of free will and our ability to change? Does this impact the way we view human responsibility for our choices?

---

2. *We can change the physical nature of our brain through our thinking and choosing.* If we can change our thinking, what does it mean to renew our minds and take every thought captive unto Christ (Rom. 12:2; 2 Cor. 10:5)?

---

3. *As we consciously direct our thinking, we can wire out toxic patterns of thinking and replace them with healthy thoughts. New thought networks grow. We increase our intelligence and bring healing to our minds and physical bodies.* If you can wire out toxic patterns of thinking and grow new, healthy thought networks, what role do your own choices play in your healing, both mentally and physically? How does this change your view of free will and your ability to choose life or death (Deut. 30:19)?

_____

_____

_____

_____

_____

_____

4. *It all starts in the realm of the mind, with our ability to think and choose—the most powerful thing in the universe after God.* If we are created in the image of God, with the ability to make choices that impact not only us but also everyone around us and the world we live in, what sense of responsibility and stewardship do you feel (Gen. 1–2)? Are you aware of how powerful your mind is?

_____

_____

_____

_____

_____

5. *Neuroplasticity, by definition, means the brain is malleable and adaptable, changing moment by moment every day.* Do you recognize how hopeful this discovery is? What does it mean to you to be able to change your mind and your life?

_____

_____

_____

_____

_____

_____

_____

6. *Scientists are finally beginning to see the brain as having renewable characteristics* (Rom. 12:2). Do you see how science and the Bible are not necessarily at odds? What do you feel about science's role in society and the Christian way of life?

_____

_____

_____

_____

_____

_____

_____

7. *Science is hovering on a precipice as we recognize the responsibility and impact of our thinking and the resultant choices we make, which have ramifications right down to the ways in which the genes of our bodies express themselves.* Now that you know more about the mind and brain, how do you feel about this responsibility? Do you see how important it is to use our minds to think on good and holy things (Phil. 4:8)? How do you see yourself starting to use your mind to make a positive impact on the world around you?

_____

_____

_____

_____

_____

_____

8. *Neurogenesis is the birth of new baby nerve cells.* How does this expand your view of God's mercy and grace? Read Lamentations 3:22–23; how do you see his mercies in light of your brain's ability to change and grow new nerve cells?

_____

_____

_____

_____

_____

_____

DISCUSSION

In light of the information in this chapter focusing on the hope that science gives us alongside Scripture, discuss the following Scriptures:

1. **Psalm 42:11 (NIV):** "Why, my soul, are you downcast? Why so disturbed within me? Put your *hope* in God, for I will yet praise him, my Savior and my God."

2. **Psalm 119:114 (NIV):** "You are my refuge and my shield; I have put my *hope* in your word."

3. **Romans 15:13 (NIV):** "May the God of *hope* fill you with all joy and peace as you trust in him, so that you may overflow with hope by the power of the Holy Spirit."

4. **Hebrews 10:23 (NIV):** "Let us hold unswervingly to the *hope* we profess, for he who promised is faithful."

5. **1 Peter 1:3 (NIV):** "Praise be to the God and Father of our Lord Jesus Christ! In his great mercy he has given us new birth into a *living hope* through the resurrection of Jesus Christ from the dead."

Write your conclusions from the discussion of these Scriptures linked to the eight scientific points above:

Mind Controls Matter

See pages 31–38 in *Switch On Your Brain*.

Main Scripture: God has not given us a spirit of fear, but of power and of *love* and of a sound mind. (2 Tim. 1:7)

Linked Science Concept: Science shows we are wired for *love* with a natural optimism bias. This means exactly what the Scripture says above.

1. *The debate in science is between the mind being what the brain does versus the brain doing the bidding of the mind.* How do you see each side of this debate in light of your faith and what you have read in *Switch On Your Brain*?

_____

_____

_____

_____

_____

_____

_____

2. *The correct view is that the mind is designed to control the body, of which the brain is a part, not the other way around.* If you can control your brain, how much responsibility and power do you have? Do you see how your thoughts can and do impact not only you but everyone and everything around you?

_____

_____

_____

_____

_____

_____

3. *Our brain does not control us; we control our brain through our thinking and choosing.* What does this mean for how we choose to think and act?

_____

_____

_____

_____

_____

_____

_____

4. *We can control our reactions to anything.* Did you ever find yourself in a situation where you knew how to react but you chose to follow your desires? How did this make you feel? What happened? Do you try to learn from such experiences and react better in the future? How do you usually try to do this?

_____

_____

_____

_____

_____

_____

_____

5. *Choices are real. You are free to make choices about how you focus your attention, and this affects how the chemicals, proteins, and wiring of your brain change and function.* Imagine the chemicals, proteins, and wiring of your brain changing as you think new thoughts. How does this make you feel? Does this knowledge empower you and encourage you to change the way you think?

_____

_____

_____

_____

_____

_____

6. *Research shows that DNA actually changes shape in response to our thoughts.* Imagine this change occurring. Do you see how powerful your thoughts are? Do you see the creative power you have in your mind, which is made in the image of the mind of Christ (1 Cor. 2:16)?

_____

_____

_____

_____

_____

_____

7. *Stress stage one is normal. Stress stage two and stage three, on the other hand, are our mind and body's response to toxic thinking— basically normal stress gone wrong.* You need to become aware of when you are stressed and how you react to stress. Think back to the last time you went through a trying situation. How did you react? Was it healthy stress or toxic stress?

---

8. Reaction *is the key word here. You cannot control the events or cir- cumstances of your life, but you can control your reactions.* Think about a recent issue you faced, and your reactions. How could you have reacted differently?

DISCUSSION

In light of the information in this chapter, discuss the following Scriptures:

1. **Isaiah 26:3 (ESV):** "You keep him in perfect peace whose mind is stayed on you, because he trusts in you."
2. **Romans 12:1–2 (ESV):** "I appeal to you therefore, brothers, by the mercies of God, to present your bodies as a living sacrifice, holy and acceptable to God, which is your spiritual worship. Do not be conformed to this world, but be transformed by the renewal of your mind, that by testing you may discern what is the will of God, what is good and acceptable and perfect."
3. **Proverbs 4:23 (ESV):** "Keep your heart with all vigilance, for from it flow the springs of life."
4. **Ephesians 4:22–24 (ESV):** "To put off your old self, which belongs to your former manner of life and is corrupt through deceitful desires, and to be renewed in the *spirit of your minds*, and to put on the new self, created after the likeness of God in true righteousness and holiness."
5. **Deuteronomy 30:19 (ESV):** "I call heaven and earth to witness against you today, that I have set before you life and death, blessing and curse. Therefore choose life, that you and your offspring may live."

Write your conclusions from the discussion of these Scriptures linked to the eight scientific points above:

23

Choice and Your Multiple-Perspective Advantage

See pages 39–54 in *Switch On Your Brain*.

Main Scripture: Let the peace (soul harmony which comes) from Christ rule (act as umpire continually) in your hearts [deciding and settling with finality all questions that arise in your minds, in that peaceful state] to which as [members of Christ's] one body you were also called [to live]. And be thankful (appreciative), [giving praise to God always]. (Col. 3:15 AMP)

Linked Science Concept: Choice is real, and free will exists. You are able to stand outside of yourself, observe your own thinking, consult with God, and change the negative, toxic thought or grow the healthy, positive thought. When you do this, your brain responds with a positive neurochemical rush and structural changes that will improve your intellect, health, and peace. You will experience soul harmony.

1. *You are not a victim. You can control your reactions. You do have a choice.* We have all been wronged at one point or another. Have you ever let a situation get to you, where you felt overwhelmed with sadness, bitterness, and hopelessness? How did this make you feel, physically and mentally? If you could go back in time to that situation, how would you choose to react?

_____

_____

_____

_____

_____

_____

_____

2. *Free will is not an illusion. Thinking it is an illusion is dangerous thinking that basically says that we are not responsible for our actions, thus providing an excuse to do whatever we want to do, with no consequences.* In light of Deuteronomy 30:19, which gives us a choice between life and death, how do you think the biblical worldview is challenged by viewing free will as an illusion? How is this dangerous?

_____

_____

_____

_____

_____

_____

_____

_____

_____

_____

3. *Our free will influences our thinking, which produces our state of mind. This is so important to human behavior and potential that I have dedicated my life to understanding the process of thought and how we can choose to think the way God wants us to think. Far from explaining away free will, neuroscientific evidence actually explains how free will works.* It is important to remember that uncertainty and human prejudice affect the way we see and interpret data in every area of academia, even science. The scientist's worldview, whether or not he or she is a Christian, will affect the way data is seen and understood. How do you view science? Why do you think you see science in this way? What influences the way you see science?

_____

_____

_____

_____

_____

_____

_____

4. *What we say and do is based on what we have already built into our minds. We evaluate this information and make our choices based on this information. Then we choose to build a new thought, and this is what drives what we say and do.* Think about your thinking. Can you recognize a pattern between your thinking and your words and actions?

_____

_____

_____

_____

_____

_____

5. *Choice has mental real estate around the front of the brain. Certain areas light up when we think and choose.* Imagine different areas lighting up as you think, speak, and act. How does this make you feel about thoughts as real things that occupy mental real estate? Do you feel you should be more careful of the way you think?

_____

_____

_____

_____

_____

_____

6. *One of the most exciting features of our frontal lobes is how they enable us, in a sense, to stand outside ourselves and observe our own thinking.* Have you ever been in a situation where you felt that you were seeing yourself do or say something, almost like watching a movie?

_____

_____

_____

_____

_____

_____

_____

7. *We have what I like to call "multiple-perspective advantage"—MPA for short. Our unique, multifaceted nature, made in God's image, allows us to see things from many different angles or perspectives.* Practice using your MPA. Think of a situation or issue you have faced. How did you use your MPA? What were the different angles or perspectives?

_____

_____

_____

_____

_____

_____

_____

8. *All of this thinking activity is real, and it can be seen on various types of brain imaging.* How does knowing thoughts are real and that we can observe our own thoughts through our words and actions change the way you view the process of thinking?

_____

_____

_____

_____

_____

_____

9. *This thinking creates signals that unzip the DNA, which then expresses genes making proteins.* Imagine this process occurring before your eyes. As you imagine, you are actually unzipping DNA and creating the roots of your words and actions! Do you see how powerful your thoughts are? Do you feel more responsibility for what you think?

_____

_____

_____

_____

_____

_____

_____

10. *We have a switch gene called the "creb gene" that we choose to switch on with our thoughts.* If you could press this switch and control your thoughts, would you? Well, you do—your thinking, feeling, and choosing control your thoughts. Do you see how your choices are that "switch"?

_____

_____

_____

_____

_____

_____

11. *Our genetic makeup fluctuates by the minute based on what we are thinking and choosing.* Our biology responds to our thinking. How does this change the way you understand Romans 12:2 and the process of renewing the mind?

_____

_____

_____

_____

_____

_____

12. *A time is coming when medical practitioners will include admonitions like Philippians 4:8 and Romans 12:2 on their prescription pads.* There are many stories of human survival and triumph in the face of extreme odds. All of those people chose to see their circumstances in a more positive light and change their attitudes. Have you experienced times in your life when positive thinking has changed the way you feel? Do you feel that a merry heart is like medicine (Prov. 17:22)? Would you recommend a good "dose" of love and joy for those suffering from physical and mental ill-health?

_____

_____

_____

_____

_____

_____

13. *From the gene myth to the truth: we are not victims of our biology; we control our biology.* How does this view of the mind empower you to make healthy decisions? Do you see how seeing yourself as a victim can lead you into a negative cycle of toxic thinking, which leads to toxic health?

_____

_____

_____

_____

_____

In light of the information in this chapter, discuss the following Scriptures:

1. **Matthew 15:11 (ESV):** "It is not what goes into the mouth that defiles a person, but what comes out of the mouth; this defiles a person."
2. **Proverbs 17:22 (ESV):** "A joyful heart is good medicine, but a crushed spirit dries up the bones."
3. **Matthew 22:37 (ESV):** "You shall love the Lord your God with all your heart and with all your soul and with all your *mind*."
4. **Isaiah 26:3 (ESV):** "You keep him in perfect peace whose *mind* is stayed on you, because he trusts in you."
5. **Colossians 3:2–5 (ESV):** "Set your *minds* on things that are above, not on things that are on earth. For you have died, and your life is hidden with Christ in God. When Christ who is your life appears, then you also will appear with him in glory. Put to death therefore what is earthly in you: sexual immorality, impurity, passion, evil desire, and covetousness, which is idolatry."

Write your conclusions from the discussion of these Scriptures linked to the thirteen scientific points above:

Your Choices Change Your Brain

See pages 55–70 in *Switch On Your Brain*.

Main Scripture: Do not conform to the pattern of this world, but be transformed by the renewing of your mind. Then you will be able to test and approve what God's will is—his good, pleasing and perfect will. (Rom. 12:2 NIV)

Linked Science Concept: Through our thoughts we can be our own micro-surgeons as we make choices that will change the circuits in our brains. We are designed to do our own brain surgery and rewire our brains by thinking and by choosing to renew our minds.

1. *Our thoughts, imagination, and choices can change the structure and function of our brains on every level: molecular, genetic, epigenetic, cellular, structural, neurochemical, electromagnetic, and even subatomic. Through our thoughts, we can be our own brain surgeons as we make choices that change the circuits in our brain. We are designed to do our own brain surgery.* Imagine you are doing thought "surgery." Do you see what you would change in your mind? Can you imagine your brain wiring changing as you make a positive choice, ridding your mind of the toxic thought? How does it make you feel that this actually happens in your brain?

2. *Choices become signals that change our brain and body, and these changes are not necessarily dictated by our genes.* If everything was controlled by our genes, how would we view free will and responsibility for our choices?

_____

_____

_____

_____

_____

_____

3. *Epigenetics is referred to as a new science, but actually it is an ancient science that we find throughout the Bible. At its most basic level, epigenetics is the fact that your thoughts and choices impact your physical brain and body, your mental health, and your spiritual development.* How do you see epigenetics in light of the biblical worldview? What does it mean to take responsibility for the consequences of our choices? If our choices can impact not only us but also the world around us, how should we view the power we have in our minds?

_____

_____

_____

_____

_____

_____

_____

_____

4. *These choices will affect not only your own spirit, soul, and body but also the people with whom you have relationships. In fact, it goes even deeper: your choices might impact the generations that follow.* If Jesus tells us to love our neighbor as ourselves, does this not apply to our neighbor of the future? If our choices affect not just us but also our children's children, how much more careful should we be about how we think, speak, and act?

_____

_____

_____

_____

_____

5. *The landmark study on agouti mice fostered a host of studies—including some done on humans—that show that not only does food change generational patterns but so does thinking.* After reading this study, do you see how good, healthy thinking, both before birth and as a child is growing up, is essential to good parenting? If you had to write a parenting book or give advice to parents, what would you say about thinking and its generational impact?

_____

_____

_____

_____

_____

6. *Taken collectively, these studies show us that the good, the bad, and the ugly do come down through the generations. But your mind is the signal—the epigenetic factor—that switches these genes on or off.* We are not victims of our biology, even if we have inherited negative traits from our ancestors. Have you ever found yourself blaming your parents or grandparents for a problem or characteristic you have? Do you recognize that you are not fated to live it out in your own life?

_____

_____

_____

_____

_____

_____

7. *Therefore, you are not destined to live out the negative patterns of your forebearers but can instead make a life choice to overcome them by tweaking their expression.* It is sometimes hard in today's world to truly believe that our thoughts are powerful. But they are! Have you ever felt trapped in family patterns of behavior? How do you feel now that you know you are not destined to live in that way?

_____

_____

_____

_____

_____

_____

8. *Epigenetic changes represent a biological response to an environmental signal. That response can be inherited through the generations via the epigenetic marks. But if you remove the signal, the epigenetic marks will fade. If you choose to add a signal, then the epigenetic marks are activated.* If this signal is our thinking, what does this mean in terms of our own free will and responsibility? Can we just blame all of our problems on our ancestors?

_____

_____

_____

_____

_____

9. *The sins of parents can create a predisposition, not a destiny. You are not responsible for something you are predisposed to because of ancestral decisions. You are responsible, however, to be aware of those predispositions, evaluate them, and make the choice to eliminate them.* How can you start changing the way you think about your past, who you are, and your family?

_____

_____

_____

_____

_____

10. *When you make a bad choice, genes switch on in the hippocampus that dampen the stress response. So God has built backup systems into our body to help us cope with life.* Have you ever made a bad choice or mistake and felt this reaction in your body? And on the flip side, have you ever been aware of how good it feels when you make a good choice?

_____

_____

_____

_____

_____

_____

_____

11. *Scientists now know that the brain has the amazing ability to reorganize moment by moment throughout life, changing its structure and function through thinking alone.* How does this make you feel? Do you see how this is God's grace, mercy, and love in action?

_____

_____

_____

_____

_____

_____

_____

12. *Neuroplasticity (the ability of the brain to change in response to thinking) can operate for you as well as against you, because whatever you think about the most will grow. This applies to both the positive and negative ends of the spectrum.* Have you ever thought about an issue so long that it made you feel depressed and hopeless? Or have you ever thought about something good that happened and felt full of joy and more inspired to do your daily tasks?

_____

_____

_____

_____

_____

_____

13. *Our perception of the environment, plus how we manage our environment, controls our bodies and lives. So if you change your perception, you change your biology. You become the master of your life instead of a victim.* How do you perceive your world? How can you change your perceptions for the better?

_____

_____

_____

_____

_____

_____

DISCUSSION

In light of the information in this chapter, discuss the following Scriptures:

1. **Deuteronomy 30:19 (ESV):** "I call heaven and earth to witness against you today, that I have set before you life and death, blessing and curse. Therefore choose life, that you and your offspring may live."
2. **Matthew 12:37 (ESV):** "For by your words you will be justified, and by your words you will be condemned."
3. **Romans 14:12 (NLT):** "Yes, each of us will give a personal account to God."
4. **Galatians 6:5 (MSG):** "Each of you must take responsibility for doing the creative best you can with your own life."
5. **Psalm 119:18 (NLT):** "Open my eyes to see the wonderful truths in your instructions."

Write your conclusions from the discussion of these Scriptures linked to the thirteen scientific points above:

Catch Those Thoughts

See pages 71–77 in *Switch On Your Brain*.

Main Scripture: We destroy arguments and every lofty opinion raised against the knowledge of God, and take every thought captive to obey Christ. (2 Cor. 10:5 ESV)

Linked Science Concept: When you objectively observe your own thinking with the view to capturing rogue thoughts, you in effect direct your attention to stop the negative impact and rewire healthy new circuits into your brain.

1. *The design of the brain allows us to capture and discipline chaotic thoughts.* How exactly does the brain's design allow us to control our thinking?

_____

_____

_____

_____

_____

_____

2. *Catching our thoughts is necessary because it calms our spirits so we can tune in and listen to God.* Have you ever felt so overwhelmed and distracted by what is going on in your life that your relationship with God took a backseat?

_____

_____

_____

_____

_____

_____

3. *When we are mindful of catching our thoughts in this way, we change our connection with God from uninvolved and independent to involved and dependent.* What do you feel like when you choose to give your problems to God instead of trying to sort them out on your own?

_____

_____

_____

_____

_____

_____

_____

4. *Research dating back to the 1970s shows that being introspectively aware of our thoughts in a disciplined way rather than letting them chaotically run rampant can bring about impressive changes in how we feel and think.* Have you experienced this in your life? How did it make you feel?

_____

_____

_____

_____

_____

_____

_____

5. *Purposefully catching your thoughts can control the brain's sensory processing, the brain's rewiring, neurotransmitters, genetic expression, and cellular activity in a positive or negative direction. You choose.* When you are in toxic situations, do you feel like you can choose how to react? Do you feel trapped? Do you now understand that you do have a choice? How does it make you feel to know you are not a prisoner of your past?

_____

_____

_____

_____

_____

6. *A chaotic mind filled with uncaptured rogue thoughts of anxiety, worry, and all manner of fear-related emotions sends out the wrong signal, right down to the level of the DNA.* Have you ever felt this in your life? Have you ever been so stressed and anxious when you think about everything that's going wrong in your life that you feel "sick to your stomach," fluey, and in pain? Do you see how negative thinking patterns can affect your biology?

_____

_____

_____

_____

_____

7. *Research has shown that five to sixteen minutes a day of focused, meditative capturing of thoughts shifts frontal brain states so that they are more likely to engage with the world, increasing the chances of a happier outlook on life.* Even with a busy life, five minutes of focused meditation is not impossible. Think of your schedule. How can you incorporate just a few minutes of healthy mind "work" into your day?

_____

_____

_____

_____

_____

_____

_____

8. *We are wired for love and we learn to fear.* What feels more normal to you, love or fear? Why do you think it feels "normal"? How does being "wired for love" relate to what the Bible says?

_____

_____

_____

_____

_____

_____

In light of the information in this chapter, discuss the following Scriptures:

1. **Romans 8:5–6 (ESV):** "For those who live according to the flesh set their minds on the things of the flesh, but those who live according to the Spirit set their minds on the things of the Spirit. For to set the mind on the flesh is death, but to set the mind on the Spirit is life and peace."

2. **1 John 4:7–8 (AMP):** "Beloved, let us [unselfishly] love and seek the best for one another, for love is from God; and everyone who loves [others] is born of God and knows God [through personal experience]. The one who does not love has not become acquainted with God [does not and never did know Him], for God is love. [He is the originator of love, and it is an enduring attribute of His nature.]"

3. **Matthew 11:28 (NLT):** "Come to me, all of you who are weary and carry heavy burdens, and I will give you rest."

4. **Philippians 4:6–7 (ESV):** "Do not be anxious about anything, but in everything by prayer and supplication with thanksgiving let your requests be made known to God. And the peace of God, which surpasses all understanding, will guard your hearts and your minds in Christ Jesus."

5. **James 4:7 (ESV):** "Submit yourselves therefore to God. Resist the devil, and he will flee from you."

Write your conclusions from the discussion of these Scriptures linked to the eight scientific points above:

_____

_____

_____

_____

_____

_____

_____

_____

_____

_____

_____

_____

_____

_____

_____

_____

KEY **5**

Entering into Directed Rest

See pages 79–92 in *Switch On Your Brain.*

Main Scripture: Be still, and know that I am God. (Ps. 46:10)

Linked Science Concept: When we direct our rest by introspection, self-reflection, and prayer; when we catch our thoughts; when we memorize and quote Scripture; and when we develop our mind intellectually, we enhance the default mode network (DMN) that improves brain function and mental, physical, and spiritual health.

1. *We have all kinds of coordinated networks in our brains that work together in an organized way, forming a constant, intrinsic chatter in the nonconscious part of our mind.* What are these networks? How does the nonconscious mind differ from the conscious mind?

_____

_____

_____

_____

_____

_____

_____

2. *Our brains maintain a high level of activity 24/7. This activity forms the brain's inner life, with the DMN dominating and becoming especially active when the mind is introspective and thinking deeply in a directed rest or idle state.* How do you feel when you think in a deep, introspective way? Do you find yourself doing this often?

_____

_____

_____

_____

_____

_____

_____

3. *As these networks function correctly, we shift into deeply introspective and meditative states that increase our intelligence and health.* What does it mean for the networks to function correctly? What stops them from functioning correctly? How can this affect our intelligence and health? How does this relate to Proverbs 23:7, which says that as a man "thinks in his heart, so is he"?

----

4. *When we switch back and forth between the various networks—for example, when we have flexible and creative thinking—we are able to shift between thoughts and capture and control them.* Have you ever experienced this type of creative thinking? How so? How did it make you feel? What happened when you thought this way? Did you get excited as ideas connected in your mind?

----

5. *When we direct our rest by introspection, self-reflection, and prayer; when we catch our thoughts; when we memorize and quote Scripture; and when we develop our mind intellectually, we accelerate the DMN and improve brain function as well as mind, body, and spiritual health.* How can you incorporate more "directed rest" moments into your life? How do you practice introspection, self-reflection, and prayer?

_____

_____

_____

_____

_____

6. *The DMN is balanced by the task positive network (TPN), which supports the active thinking required for making decisions. The more balanced we are, the more wisdom we apply in our thinking and decisions. This action step of the TPN is necessary for effective brain and mind change.* Is your thinking balanced or toxic? How does this affect your wisdom? When you are unbalanced, and your life feels like it is falling apart, what kind of decisions do you tend to make?

_____

_____

_____

_____

_____

7. *Miswiring of brain regions involved in the DMN, which leads to all kinds of ups and downs in the DMN, may even be part of mind issues ranging from Alzheimer's to schizophrenia.* When you are worried, anxious, fearful, and so forth, do you feel as if your mind is going crazy and out of control? Do you forget tasks or lose concentration?

_____

_____

_____

_____

_____

_____

8. *Toxic thinking produces this miswiring, which causes increased activity in the DMN, resulting in a decrease of activity in the TPN. This causes maladaptive, depressive ruminations and a decrease in the ability to solve problems. This makes us feel foggy, confused, negative, and depressed.* Think of a time when this happened to you recently. How could you have reacted differently?

_____

_____

_____

_____

_____

_____

9. *Your mind can powerfully and unexpectedly change your brain in positive ways when you intentionally direct your attention—and the same applies in the negative direction. This is called the plastic paradox.* How do you see this in light of "bringing every thought into captivity to the obedience of Christ" (2 Cor. 10:5) and "renewing . . . your mind" (Rom. 12:2)?

DISCUSSION

In light of the information in this chapter, discuss the following Scriptures:

1. **Mark 6:31 (AMP):** "He said to them, 'Come away by yourselves to a secluded place and rest a little while'—for there were many [people who were continually] coming and going, and they could not even find time to eat."

2. **Proverbs 3:5–6 (ESV):** "Trust in the LORD with all your heart, and do not lean on your own understanding. In all your ways acknowledge him, and he will make straight your paths."

3. **Isaiah 26:3 (NIV):** "You will keep in perfect peace those whose minds are steadfast, because they trust in you."

4. **Proverbs 4:23 (NIV):** "Above all else, guard your heart, for everything you do flows from it."

5. **Proverbs 1:7 (ESV):** "The fear of the LORD is the beginning of knowledge; fools despise wisdom and instruction."

Write your conclusions from the discussion of these Scriptures linked to the nine scientific points above:

Stop Milkshake-Multitasking

See pages 93–102 in *Switch On Your Brain*.

Main Scripture: Dear friend, listen well to my words; tune your ears to my voice. Keep my message in plain view at all times. Concentrate! Learn it by heart! Those who discover these words live, really live; body and soul, they're bursting with health. Keep vigilant watch over your heart; that's where life starts. (Prov. 4:20–23 MSG)

Linked Science Concept: Multitasking is a persistent myth. Paying deep, focused attention to one task at a time is the correct way.

1. *The truth about multitasking is that it is a persistent myth.* What do you think about multitasking? What have you heard or read about multitasking?

_____

_____

_____

_____

_____

_____

2. *What we really do is shift our attention rapidly and haphazardly from task to task, resulting in two negative things: (1) We don't devote as much focused attention as we should to a specific activity, task, or piece of information, and (2) we sacrifice the quality of our attention. I call this milkshake-multitasking.* Are you guilty of milkshake-multitasking? When you try to do multiple tasks at once, what happens? How do you feel?

_____

_____

_____

_____

_____

_____

3. *This milkshake-multitasking creates patterns of flightiness and a lack of concentration that unfortunately are often erroneously labeled ADD and ADHD—which are not real scientific disorders. Too often this results in unnecessary medication, which adds fuel to the fire.* Have you ever experienced this in your life, or know someone who has? How do you see ADD and ADHD and multitasking?

_____

_____

_____

_____

_____

_____

4. *The general pattern today is that so much attention is paid to tweeting, Instagramming, and Facebooking that we forget all about enjoying the moment.* Do you feel that too much time on social media has decreased your attention span and ability to focus? Do you know people who experience this?

_____

_____

_____

_____

_____

_____

5. *So-called social media experts tell us that information needs to be provided in bite-size amounts and in a constant stream of new information before the previous information has even been digested. This is not stimulation; it is bombardment.* Do you ever feel overwhelmed by the amount and rate of information we have access to in today's world? How does this affect your ability to think and concentrate?

----

6. *Milkshake-multitasking decreases our attention and makes us increasingly less able to focus on our thought habits. This opens us up to shallow and weak judgments and decisions, and it results in passive mindlessness.* Have you ever made a bad decision when you were trying to do too many things at once? Have you ever agreed to do or say something when you were busy doing something else? How "wise" were your decisions or words?

----

7. *Scientists are seeing the evidence of deep, intellectual thought versus milkshake-multitasking in the brain.* How does this relate to what the Bible teaches about thinking?

8. *I saw the greatest changes in patients who willfully, determinedly, and persistently chose to focus their attention on improving their skills and restoring function.* Have you ever been desperate to change the way you think? Do you understand that it will take persistence, determination, and discipline? Do you feel like you can do this? How do you see your own strength and abilities? How does this relate to what God promises?

In light of the information in this chapter, discuss the following Scriptures:

1. **Romans 12:12 (NIV):** "Be joyful in hope, patient in affliction, faithful in prayer."

2. **Galatians 6:9 (ESV):** "And let us not grow weary of doing good, for in due season we will reap, if we do not give up."

3. **Luke 10:38–42 (AMP):** "Now while they were on their way, Jesus entered a village [called Bethany], and a woman named Martha welcomed Him into her home. She had a sister named Mary, who seated herself at the Lord's feet and was continually listening to His teaching. But Martha was very busy and distracted with all of her serving responsibilities; and she approached Him and said, "Lord, is it of no concern to You that my sister has left me to do the serving alone? Tell her to help me and do her part." But the Lord replied to her, "Martha, Martha, you are worried and bothered and anxious about so many things; but only one thing is necessary, for Mary has chosen the good part [that which is to her advantage], which will not be taken away from her.""

4. **Colossians 3:23–24 (ESV):** "Whatever you do, work heartily, as for the Lord and not for men, knowing that from the Lord you will receive the inheritance as your reward. You are serving the Lord Christ."

5. **1 Corinthians 14:33 (ESV):** "For God is not a God of confusion but of peace."

Write your conclusions from the discussion of these Scriptures linked to the eight scientific points above:

Thinking, God, and the Quantum Physics Brain

See pages 103–22 in *Switch On Your Brain*.

Main Scripture: Today I have given you the choice between life and death, between blessings and curses. Now I call on heaven and earth to witness the choice you make. Oh, that you would choose life, so that you and your descendants might live! (Deut. 30:19 NLT)

Linked Science Concepts: The process of thinking and choosing is the most powerful thing in the universe after God, and it is a phenomenal gift from God to be treasured and used properly. The basic ingredients of quantum physics are: paying attention, thinking and choosing, and consequence.

1. *There is the sensory world of our five senses, there is the world of electromagnetism and the atom, and then there is the deeper quantum world that is fundamental to the other worlds.* How does the quantum world differ from the worlds of the senses and atoms?

_____

_____

_____

_____

_____

_____

2. *This quantum world challenges physicists' perception of linear time, orderly space, and fixed realities and it turns on its head the Cartesian Newtonian world that sees humans as machines with exchangeable parts.* How does the quantum world challenge the view that humans are just machines? How does this relate to the way the Bible views humankind?

_____

_____

_____

_____

_____

_____

3. *Quantum physics, which is different from classical physics, is a way of explaining how the things that make up atoms work and making sense of how the smallest things in nature work.* What is classical physics? Did you assume that it was the only kind of physics? If it were the only kind of physics, how would that change the way we view reality?

_____

_____

_____

_____

_____

_____

4. Quantum *means energy, so quantum physics also tells us how electromagnetic waves—like light waves—work.* What do you know about light waves and energy?

_____

_____

_____

_____

_____

_____

5. *Quantum mechanics is the mathematical framework used to describe this energy and how it works.* Do you see how science, and even mathematics, is a description of God's creation?

_____

_____

_____

_____

_____

_____

_____

_____

6. *Quantum physics basically says:*

- *your consciousness affects the behaviors of subatomic particles,*
- *particles move backward and forward in time and appear in all possible places at once, and*
- *the universe is connected with faster-than-light transfers of information.*

What do each of these points essentially mean? How do they differ from classical physics? What does this mean to you and in your life?

_____

_____

_____

_____

_____

----

7. *Five main ideas are presented in quantum theory:*

- *Energy is not a continuous stream but comes in small, discrete units.*
- *The basic units behave both like particles and like waves.*
- *The movement of these particles is random.*
- *It is physically impossible to know both the position and the momentum of a particle at the same time.*
- *The atomic world is nothing like the world we live in.*

How do these ideas change the way you view science and reality? How do you understand what is "real"?

----

8. *Quantum theory converts science's conception of humans from being mere cogs in a gigantic, mechanical machine to being freethinking agents whose conscious, free choices affect the physical world. This is called the observer effect.* How do you understand this in light of what the Bible teaches?

_____

_____

_____

_____

_____

_____

_____

9. *The Copenhagen interpretation of quantum theory says that the particle is what you measure it to be. This means our perceptions determine the outcome; we perceive the world through the thoughts (memories) we have built into our brains.* What have you implanted in your brain? Are they life-giving mindsets, or toxic ones? How do you see them affecting your reality?

_____

_____

_____

_____

_____

_____

10. *The Quantum Zeno Effect (QZE) is the repeated effort that causes learning to take place.* Do you often feel that change should happen immediately? Do you recognize and understand that true change takes time and effort?

11. *The law of entanglement in quantum physics states that relationship is the defining characteristic of everything in space and time. Because of the pervasive nature of the entanglement of atomic particles, relationship is independent of distance and requires no physical link. Everything and everyone is linked, and we all affect each other.* If all of us are entangled in each other's lives, how important are your choices?

12. *Thought signals seem to move faster than the speed of light and in ways that classical physics cannot explain. This means our mind controls matter and is therefore a creative force.* How does this change the way you view 1 Corinthians 2:16, where it says we "have the mind of Christ"?

_____

_____

_____

_____

_____

13. *Humans are seen as observers who exert an effect that is unpredictable. And it is not just humans who are unpredictable. The unpredictability reaches down to the level of electrons and photons of light, which cannot have a definite momentum or position at the same time; particles are neither particles nor waves because they are both. And as for quarks, bosons, and now preons and strings—they are simply nothing that is all over the place!* Do you see how powerful and unpredictable free will is? How important is forgiveness and perseverance in a universe where everyone is free to choose?

_____

_____

_____

_____

_____

14. *The random and unpredictable nature of quantum physics is called the Heisenberg uncertainty principle. This principle is a way God shows us that we do not control the future. He does.* How do you feel about giving God control of your thinking and your life?

_____

_____

_____

_____

_____

_____

_____

15. *Quantum physics math prediction is all about mathematically showing this uncertainty, which basically undergirds free will.* Do you feel that many people dislike the idea that they do not control or fully understand the world around them? Why?

_____

_____

_____

_____

_____

_____

_____

16. *I believe God is taking us through the material world into the spiritual world to get to know him more deeply, and the quantum concept is part of this journey.* How has learning about quantum physics enabled you to get to know God and his world better? How do you think it will help you to strengthen your relationship with God?

_____

_____

_____

_____

_____

_____

_____

_____

DISCUSSION

In light of the information in this chapter, discuss the following Scriptures:

1. **John 1:1–5 (AMP):** "In the beginning [before all time] was the Word (Christ), and the Word was with God, and the Word was God Himself. He was [continually existing] in the beginning [co-eternally] with God. All things were made and came into existence through Him; and without Him not even one thing was made that has come into being. In Him was life [and the power to bestow life], and the life was the Light of men. The Light shines on in the darkness, and the darkness did not understand it or overpower it or appropriate it or absorb it [and is unreceptive to it]."

2. **1 Corinthians 2:16 (NLT):** "For, 'Who can know the LORD's thoughts? Who knows enough to teach him?' But we understand these things, for we have the mind of Christ."

3. **Matthew 6:25–34 (ESV):** "Therefore I tell you, do not be anxious about your life, what you will eat or what you will drink, nor about your body, what you will put on. Is not life more than food, and the body more than clothing? Look at the birds of the air: they neither sow nor reap nor gather into barns, and yet your heavenly Father feeds them. Are you not of more value than they? And which of you by being anxious can add a single hour to his span of life? And why are you anxious about clothing? Consider the lilies of the field, how they grow: they neither toil nor spin, yet I tell you, even Solomon in all his glory was not arrayed like one of these."

4. **Jeremiah 29:11 (ESV):** "For I know the plans I have for you, declares the LORD, plans for welfare and not for evil, to give you a future and a hope."

5. **Psalm 115:3 (NLT):** "Our God is in the heavens, and he does as he wishes."

Write your conclusions from the discussion of these Scriptures linked to the sixteen scientific points above:

_____

_____

_____

_____

_____

_____

_____

_____

_____

_____

_____

_____

_____

_____

_____

_____

The Science of Thought

See pages 123–35 in *Switch On Your Brain.*

Main Scripture: Therefore put away all filthiness and rampant wickedness and receive with meekness the implanted word, which is able to save your souls. (James 1:21 ESV)

Linked Science Concept: What you wire into your brain through thinking impacts the effectiveness of your life. The nonconscious mind is where up to 90–99.9 percent of our activity is. It is the root level that stores the thoughts with the emotions and perceptions, and it impacts the conscious mind and what we say and do. Everything is first a thought. The Geodesic Information Processing Theory is a scientific way of understanding this.

1. *The Geodesic Information Processing Theory deals with the science of thought. It is a description of how we think, choose, and build thoughts and the impact of this on our brain and behavior.* How does this theory work? How did you see the process of thinking before you read this book?

_____

_____

_____

_____

_____

_____

_____

2. *I show in my Geodesic Information Processing Theory that the brain works in neurological pillars and multiple parallel circuits, which means there is a lot of interconnectivity among the networks of the brain.* How does this differ from the core traditional left brain/right brain way of understanding thinking?

_____

_____

_____

_____

_____

_____

_____

3. *It is our choices that make something out of nothing. It is our choices that collapse the probabilities into actualities that define the state of our metacognition, which, in turn, inform our cognition and symbolic actions.* Can you think of a time or a situation when your choices made something into a reality?

_____

_____

_____

_____

_____

_____

4. *My Switch On Your Brain 21-Day Brain Detox Plan, which is based on my theory and research, is designed to help improve your thinking and choices and subsequent happiness and health.* How does the program work? What are the principles behind the program?

_____

_____

_____

_____

_____

_____

5. *It is our choices that either create healthy thought universes in our brain or turn the powerless lie into a toxic thought universe—which is essentially evil. This is the incredible power God has given us: to be able to think and choose and create reality. This reality can be good or evil, based on our choices.* How do you see this in light of Deuteronomy 30:19, which tells us we can choose life or death, and in light of Jesus's call for us to follow him in the Gospels?

_____

_____

_____

_____

_____

6. *After a period of repeated thinking about the choice over two to three cycles of twenty-one days, the new thought moves into the nonconscious metacognitive level, where it becomes part of our internal perception. This process is called* automatization *and becomes part of your belief system, shaping and influencing your choices.* What kinds of things have you been thinking about a lot lately? Do you want these kinds of thoughts to shape the way you see life? What would you prefer to have in your mind? Remember, whatever you think about the most will grow!

_____

_____

_____

_____

_____

7. *Everything you do and say is first a thought.* Think back to something you did or said recently. What was the thought or thoughts that led to that action? Can you recognize how you got from the thought to the action?

_____

_____

_____

_____

_____

_____

8. *The nonconscious metacognitive mind is filled with the thoughts you have been building since you were born, and they form the perceptual base from which you see life.* These thoughts act, in a way, like glasses, shaping the way you view the world. How do you see the world? What thoughts have created your worldview? How do they align with what the Bible says?

_____

_____

_____

_____

_____

_____

In light of the information in this chapter, discuss the following Scriptures:

1. **Ecclesiastes 3:1–5 (ESV):** "For everything there is a season, and a time for every matter under heaven: a time to be born, and a time to die; a time to plant, and a time to pluck up what is planted; a time to kill, and a time to heal; a time to break down, and a time to build up; a time to weep, and a time to laugh; a time to mourn, and a time to dance; a time to cast away stones, and a time to gather stones together; a time to embrace, and a time to refrain from embracing."

2. **Ephesians 1:10 (ESV):** "As a plan for the fullness of time, to unite all things in him, things in heaven and things on earth."

3. **1 Corinthians 6:12 (NIV):** "'I have the right to do anything,' you say—but not everything is beneficial."

4. **Proverbs 16:3 (NIV):** "Commit to the LORD whatever you do, and he will establish your plans."

5. **Revelation 3:20 (ESV):** "Behold, I stand at the door and knock. If anyone hears my voice and opens the door, I will come in to him and eat with him, and he with me."

Write your conclusions from the discussion of these Scriptures linked to the eight scientific points above:

....

....

The 21-Day Brain Detox

See pages 139–201 in *Switch On Your Brain*.

Each day it will take around seven to ten minutes to complete the five steps of the program: *Gather, Focused Reflection, Write, Revisit,* and *Active Reach*, which are described in further detail in *Switch On Your Brain* and my online program (www.21daybraindetox.com).

We all have busy lives, with many demands on our time. This detox program was specifically created with those demands in mind, and can easily be incorporated into your daily routine as it takes just seven minutes a day—I do my detox each morning as I am getting ready, so I have made it part of my lifestyle. It will help you deal with the issues you face in your life, and is based on an understanding of the information in *Switch On Your Brain* and this workbook.

What Do You Do?

1. You do the five steps of the *Switch On Your Brain* technique daily for twenty-one days on **one** specific toxic thought that the Holy Spirit has revealed to you through prayer.

2. You stick with this one thought for sixty-three days (three cycles of twenty-one days)—one cycle builds the thought into a long term memory; the next two cycles turn the new thought into a habit. When you have finished this, you start the next sixty-three days with a new thought.

3. It takes you seven to ten minutes to work through the five steps each day, and then you do your selected *active reach* at least seven times throughout the day. So the active reach, step 5, has an action component that you *do* throughout the day. You have worked out what your active reach will be through using the insight you gained from steps 1–4. The active reach can be as short as one to seven seconds or up to one minute each. So your practice time can be as little as seven seconds up to seven minutes a day total. You can do active reaches for longer, if you wish, but not too much longer.

4. One brain detox cycle is sixty-three days total.

5. One sixty-three day cycle is often enough time to deal with an issue, but repeat the cycle as many times as you feel is necessary to eliminate the toxicity, especially since some issues are deeper seated than others.

6. Remember: you are simultaneously breaking down a toxic thought and building up a healthy thought.

7. You need to practice automatizing the new healthy thought by consciously using it for at least two more twenty-one-day cycles.

LEARNING: Read the above seven-step process three times out loud; explain it to yourself three times; write the process down three times; practice saying it three times to yourself without looking; now explain the seven steps to someone. It is important that you learn these steps by heart to help you use them as effectively as possible. Here's how:

The Five Steps

Let's dive deeper into the five steps. Simply put, they are:

Gather

Focused Reflection

Write

Revisit

Active Reach

1. Gather

The *gather* step is all about becoming aware of all the signals that are coming into your mind from the external environment through the five senses and understanding the internal environment of your mind.

QUESTION: What are you experiencing through your five senses as you are reading this? Try to describe this in as much detail as possible. This is a simple exercise just to help you become aware of what is coming into your mind. This simple awareness can be developed to the point where you learn not to let any thought go through your mind unchecked.

_____

_____

_____

_____

_____

QUESTION: What thoughts are bubbling up into your conscious mind from your nonconscious mind at this moment? How many? Write them down.

_____

_____

_____

_____

QUESTION: Can you determine the attitude of the thoughts that are currently moving through your conscious mind? Try to focus in on the feelings they are generating and describe them in as much detail as possible. How does your mind feel? How does your body feel?

_____

_____

_____

_____

_____

QUESTION: Do the thoughts in your conscious mind at this moment make you feel peaceful or worried? Be aware of how your body feels. Are you tensing your shoulders? Is there an adrenaline rush going through your body?

_____

_____

_____

_____

_____

QUESTION: Do you feel like a victim of or a victor over what is swarming through your mind at the moment from the external and internal signals?

_____

_____

_____

_____

_____

_____

QUESTION: Did you know you are able to accept or reject the thoughts flowing through your mind? How does this make you feel? What are you going to do about this from now on?

_____

_____

_____

_____

_____

_____

QUESTION: You do not have to be dominated by your perceptual library—in other words, your emotions. Do you feel dominated by your feelings that have arisen out of the thoughts active in your mind?

_____

_____

_____

_____

_____

_____

QUESTION: Ask yourself, "Do I want this information to be a part of me?" What would you rather have a part of you? Why?

_____

_____

_____

_____

_____

_____

_____

_____

_____

QUESTION: Toxic thoughts are the result of bad choices. Stress stages two and three are your body's reaction to toxic thoughts. Can you feel the stress reaction—heart pounding, adrenaline pumping, or muscles tensing up in your body?

_____

_____

_____

_____

_____

_____

_____

_____

2. Focused Reflection

Focused reflection is a targeted and deliberate way of thinking that is disciplined, intellectual, and characterized by attention regulation, body awareness, emotion regulation, and a sense of self that changes the brain positively.

QUESTION: Now that you are aware that thoughts are unstable and changeable when they are in your conscious cognitive mind, can you focus on one in particular and start experimenting with changing it?

_____

_____

_____

_____

_____

_____

QUESTION: You have to make a decision. Do you want to build memories out of this new information coming into your mind? How can you improve your memories?

_____

_____

_____

_____

_____

_____

QUESTION: Have you ever found yourself rehearsing something over and over for days on end, almost like you couldn't get it out of your head? How did that make you feel?

_____

_____

_____

_____

_____

_____

QUESTION: How do you think you can tear down the toxic stronghold?

_____

_____

_____

_____

_____

_____

QUESTION: What role does the heart play in focused reflection?

_____

_____

_____

_____

_____

_____

3. Write

Writing down your thoughts is important in the *Switch On Your Brain* technique because the actual process of writing consolidates the memory and adds clarity to what you have been thinking about. It helps you better see the area that needs to be detoxed by allowing you to perceive your nonconscious and conscious thoughts in a visual way. It is almost like putting your brain on paper.

QUESTION: What does writing do to help your detoxing?

_____

_____

_____

_____

_____

_____

_____

QUESTION: What do the basal ganglia help with?

_____

_____

_____

_____

_____

_____

QUESTION: What happens in your brain when you write things down?

QUESTION: How should you write down your thoughts?

QUESTION: Why should you pour your thoughts out?

4. Revisit

Revisiting what you have written will be a revealing process. This is exciting as well, because it is a progressive "moving-forward" step; you revisit where you are and look at how to make change happen.

QUESTION: How can thoughts be redesigned?

_____

_____

_____

_____

_____

_____

_____

_____

QUESTION: What is the main purpose of this self-reflection?

_____

_____

_____

_____

_____

_____

_____

_____

QUESTION: Why is it important to think through your reactions again, evaluate the toxicity levels, and retranscribe them?

_____

_____

_____

_____

_____

_____

_____

_____

QUESTION: What does it mean to you to evaluate where you have come from and where you are going?

_____

_____

_____

_____

_____

_____

_____

_____

_____

5. Active Reach

Active reaches are the challenging but fun part of this plan because they are actions and exercises you say and/or do during the course of the day and evening. You, in essence, are practicing the new healthy thought until it becomes automatized like a good habit.

QUESTION: What is the power of the *doing* nature of this active reach step?

_____

_____

_____

_____

_____

_____

_____

QUESTION: How does your faith manifest? Work out some ideas for active reaches that will help your faith grow.

_____

_____

_____

_____

_____

_____

QUESTION: How does active reaching help you feel truth?

21-Day Detox Worksheet Example

1. Gather (1–2 minutes)

   Purpose: bring a toxic thought into consciousness. As you identify the toxic thought in the breaking-down process, you immediately, prayerfully, and consciously think of a replacement thought.

   Activity:

   _____

   _____

   _____

   _____

   _____

   _____

   _____

   _____

   _____

2. Focused Reflection (1–2 minutes)

Purpose: loosen up toxic branches. Now, grow and integrate healthy branches by reflecting on the positive replacement thought for that branch. Don't dwell on the negative because it will grow: focus on what you are replacing the negative with.

Activity:

_____

_____

_____

_____

_____

_____

3. Writing (1–2 minutes)

Purpose: start shaking the branches to loosen the glue and remove the energy from the toxic thought so it can die. Add more information and link with other branches by writing the positive alongside the negative.

Activity:

_____

_____

_____

_____

_____

_____

4. Revisit (1–2 minutes)

Purpose: shift the glue and energy to the new healthy thought. You are doing the same thing in the breaking-down and building-up processes here. The steps cross over because you are planning the solution to replace the problem. This starts stabilizing the branches to firm up the "glue" bonds.

Activity:

_____

_____

_____

_____

_____

_____

5. Active Reach (1–2 minutes)

Purpose: start melting down the branches. This is the same step as in the breaking-down process, but here you actually finalize, plan, and *do* the active reaches. This strengthens the new thought branches and builds the long-term memory into a habit over time.

Activity:

_____

_____

_____

_____

_____

_____

Conclusion

Congratulations! You have completed the *Switch On Your Brain Workbook* and are on your way to becoming *happier, healthier in your mind and body, more prosperous, and more intelligent.* You have begun the process of choosing to renew your mind, but remember this is a daily task!

This workbook supplements the 21-Day Brain Detox™ program found in my book *Switch On Your Brain* and online at 21daybraindetox.com. As I mentioned in the book, this program is based on the principles of neuroplasticity (that the brain can change as a result of thinking) and neurogenesis (the birth of new brain cells daily). The program length is twenty-one days, since it takes around twenty-one days to rewire neural pathways and begin building a new way of thinking about your life, plus forty-two more days (another two sets of twenty-one days, for a total of sixty-three days) to establish a new habit. So twenty-one days to build a long-term memory and another two cycles of twenty-one days to turn the new memory into a habit. I recommend you repeat the twenty-one-day program found in *Switch On Your Brain* three times per issue or problem you face for the rest of your life, so this is essentially a scientific technique for renewing the mind.

The "talk" between the conscious and nonconscious mind discussed in the book and workbook requires discipline and practice, but if you put the program tips into action for just seven minutes a day, within three weeks you will have removed a toxic thinking habit and built a new way of thinking about the issues and difficulties you face—through your choices and perseverance! And in another forty-two days you will have automatized this to a point where it meaningfully impacts your daily life.

Although this process may sound daunting, it is simple and easy to apply in your everyday life. And once you have developed a pattern of renewing your mind, it becomes easier to do—almost like second nature! The hard work you put in when starting the 21-Day Brain Detox will positively affect the way you live your life and truly enable you to offer yourself as a "living sacrifice"—body, mind, and spirit—every day for the rest of your life (Rom. 12:1–2).

Happy thinking, and happy living!

Recommended Reading

Science/Philosophy

Breggin, Peter Roger. *Brain-Disabling Treatments in Psychiatry: Drugs, Electroshock, and the Psychopharmaceutical Complex*. New York: Springer, 2008.

———. *Toxic Psychiatry: Why Therapy, Empathy, and Love Must Replace the Drugs, Electroshock, and Biochemical Theories of the "New Psychiatry."* New York: St. Martin's Press, 1991.

Breggin, Peter Roger, and David Cohen. *Your Drug May Be Your Problem: How and Why to Stop Taking Psychiatric Medications*. Philadelphia: DaCapo Life Long, 2007.

Caplan, Paula J. *They Say You're Crazy: How the World's Most Powerful Psychiatrists Decide Who's Normal*. Reading: Addison-Wesley, 1995.

Clayton, Philip. *Mind and Emergence: From Quantum to Consciousness*. Oxford: Oxford University Press, 2004.

Gøtzsche, Peter C. *Deadly Medicines and Organised Crime: How Big Pharma Has Corrupted Healthcare*. London: Radcliffe, 2013.

Healy, David. *Pharmageddon*. Berkeley: University of California Press, 2012.

Kelly, Edward F. *Irreducible Mind: Toward a Psychology for the 21st Century*. Lanham: Rowman & Littlefield, 2007.

Kelly, Edward F., Adam Crabtree, and Paul Marshall. *Beyond Physicalism: Toward Reconciliation of Science and Spirituality*. Lanham: Rowman & Littlefield, 2015.

Kinderman, Peter. *The New Laws of Psychology*. London: Constable & Robinson Ltd., 2014.

———. *A Prescription for Psychiatry: Why We Need a Whole New Approach to Mental Health and Wellbeing*. New York: Palgrave Macmillan, 2014.

Kinderman, P., M. Schwannauer, E. Pontin, and S. Tai. "Psychological Processes Mediate the Impact of Familial Risk, Social Circumstances and Life Events on Mental Health." *PLoS One* 8 (2013): e76564.

Moncrieff, Joanna. *The Myth of the Chemical Cure: A Critique of Psychiatric Drug Treatment*. New York: Palgrave Macmillan, 2008.

———. "The Nature of Mental Disorder: Disease, Distress, or Personal Tendency?" *Philosophy, Psychiatry & Psychology* 21, no. 3 (2014): 257–60.

Nagel, Thomas. *Mind and Cosmos: Why the Materialist Neo-Darwinian Conception of Nature Is Almost Certainly False*. New York: Oxford University Press, 2012.

Peele, Stanton. *Diseasing of America: Addiction Treatment Out of Control*. Lexington: Lexington Books, 1989.

Peele, Stanton, and Archie Brodsky. *Love and Addiction*. Watertown: Broadrow Publications, 2015.

Penrose, Roger. *The Emperor's New Mind: Concerning Computers, Minds, and the Laws of Physics*. Oxford: Oxford University Press, 1989.

———. *Shadows of the Mind: A Search for the Missing Science of Consciousness*. Oxford: Oxford University Press, 1994.

Polkinghorne, J. C. *The Quantum World*. London: Longman, 1984.

———. *Quantum Theory: A Very Short Introduction*. Oxford: Oxford University Press, 2002.

Popper, Karl R., and John C. Eccles. *The Self and Its Brain*. New York: Springer International, 1977.

Rapley, Mark, Joanna Moncrieff, and Jaqui Dillon, eds. *De-Medicalizing Misery: Psychiatry, Psychology and the Human Condition*. New York: Palgrave Macmillan, 2011.

Satel, Sally L., and Scott O. Lilienfeld. *Brainwashed: The Seductive Appeal of Mindless Neuroscience*. New York: Basic Books, 2013.

Schwartz, Jeffrey, and Sharon Begley. *The Mind and the Brain: Neuroplasticity and the Power of Mental Force*. New York: Regan Books/HarperCollins, 2002.

Sommers, Christina Hoff, and Sally L. Satel. *One Nation Under Therapy: How the Helping Culture Is Eroding Self-Reliance*. New York: St. Martin's Press, 2005.

Stapp, Henry P. *Mind, Matter, and Quantum Mechanics*. Berlin: Springer-Verlag, 1993.

———. *Mindful Universe: Quantum Mechanics and the Participating Observer*. Berlin: Springer, 2007.

———. *Quantum Mechanical Theories of Consciousness*. Berkeley: Lawrence Berkeley National Laboratory, 2004.

Thomas, Philip, Patience Seebohm, Jan Wallcraft, Jayasree Kalathil, and Suman Fernando. "Personal Consequences of the Diagnosis of Schizophrenia: A Preliminary Report from the Inquiry into the Schizophrenia Label." *Mental Health and Social Inclusion* 17, no. 3 (2013): 135–39.

Torey, Zoltan. *The Crucible of Consciousness: An Integrated Theory of Mind and Brain*. Cambridge: MIT Press, 2009.

Uttal, William R. *The New Phrenology: The Limits of Localizing Cognitive Processes in the Brain*. Cambridge: MIT Press, 2001.

Whitaker, Robert. *Anatomy of an Epidemic: Magic Bullets, Psychiatric Drugs, and the Astonishing Rise of Mental Illness in America*. New York: Crown Publishers, 2010.

Theology/Philosophy

Keener, Craig S. *The Mind of the Spirit: Paul's Approach to Transformed Thinking*. Grand Rapids: Baker Academic, 2016.

McGrath, Alister E. *Dawkins' God: Genes, Memes, and the Meaning of Life*. Malden: Blackwell Pub., 2005.

——. *A Fine-Tuned Universe: The Quest for God in Science and Theology (the 2009 Gifford Lectures)*. Louisville: Westminster John Knox Press, 2009.

——. *The Science of God: An Introduction to Scientific Theology*. Grand Rapids: Eerdmans, 2004.

——. *The Twilight of Atheism: The Rise and Fall of Disbelief in the Modern World*. New York: Doubleday, 2004.

McGrath, Alister E., and Joanna Collicutt McGrath. *The Dawkins Delusion: Atheist Fundamentalism and the Denial of the Divine*. Downers Grove: InterVarsity Press, 2007.

Middleton, J. Richard. *The Liberating Image: The Imago Dei in Genesis 1*. Grand Rapids: Brazos Press, 2005.

——. *A New Heaven and a New Earth: Reclaiming Biblical Eschatology*. Grand Rapids: Baker Academic, 2014.

Plantinga, Alvin. *Where the Conflict Really Lies: Science, Religion, and Naturalism*. New York: Oxford University Press, 2011.

——. *Knowledge and Christian Belief*. Grand Rapids: Eerdmans, 2015.

Plantinga, Alvin, and Nicholas Wolterstorff. *Faith and Rationality: Reason and Belief in God*. Notre Dame: University of Notre Dame Press, 1983.

Plantinga, Alvin, Kelly James Clark, and Michael C. Rea. *Reason, Metaphysics, and Mind: New Essays on the Philosophy of Alvin Plantinga*. New York: Oxford University Press, 2012.

Polkinghorne, J. C. *Belief in God in an Age of Science*. New Haven: Yale University Press, 1998.

——. *Exploring Reality: The Intertwining of Science and Religion*. New Haven: Yale University Press, 2005.

——. *Meaning in Mathematics*. Oxford: Oxford University Press, 2011.

——. *Quantum Physics and Theology: An Unexpected Kinship*. New Haven: Yale University Press, 2007.

——. *Quarks, Chaos & Christianity: Questions to Science and Religion*. New York: Crossroads, 1996.

———. *Science and Creation: The Search for Understanding*. Philadelphia: Templeton Foundation Press, 2006.

———. *Science and Religion in Quest of Truth*. New Haven: Yale University Press, 2011.

———. *The Trinity and an Entangled World: Relationality in Physical Science and Theology*. Grand Rapids: Eerdmans, 2010.

———. *The Work of Love: Creation As Kenosis*. Grand Rapids: Eerdmans, 2001.

Swinburne, Richard. *The Coherence of Theism*. Oxford: Clarendon Press, 1993.

———. *The Evolution of the Soul*. Oxford: Clarendon Press, 1986.

———. *Faith and Reason*. Oxford: Clarendon Press, 2005.

———. *Free Will and Modern Science*. Oxford: Oxford University Press, 2011.

Swinburne, Richard, Lynne Rudder Baker, William Jaworski, James K. Dew, and David P. Hunt. "Précis of 'Mind, Brain, and Free Will.'" *European Journal for Philosophy of Religion* (2014): 1–63.

Swinburne, Richard, and Alan G. Padgett. *Reason and the Christian Religion: Essays in Honour of Richard Swinburne*. Oxford: Clarendon Press, 1994.

Ward, Keith. *The Big Questions in Science and Religion*. West Conshohocken, PA: Templeton Foundation Press, 2008.

———. *Christ and the Cosmos: A Reformulation of Trinitarian Doctrine*. Cambridge: Cambridge University Press, 2015.

———. *God, Faith & the New Millennium: Christian Belief in an Age of Science*. Oxford: Oneworld, 1998.

———. *Morality, Autonomy, and God*. London: Oneworld, 2013.

———. *Pascal's Fire: Scientific Faith and Religious Understanding*. Oxford: Oneworld, 2006.

———. *Religion and Community*. Oxford: Clarendon Press, 2000.

———. *Religion and Creation*. New York: Oxford University Press, 1996.

Wright, N. T. *After You Believe: Why Christian Character Matters*. New York: HarperOne, 2010.

———. *The Climax of the Covenant: Christ and the Law in Pauline Theology*. Minneapolis: Fortress Press, 1992.

———. *Evil and the Justice of God*. Downers Grove, IL: InterVarsity Press, 2006.

———. *How God Became King: The Forgotten Story of the Gospels*. New York: HarperOne, 2012.

———. *The Kingdom New Testament: A Contemporary Translation*. New York: HarperOne, 2011.

———. *Surprised by Hope: Rethinking Heaven, the Resurrection, and the Mission of the Church*. New York: HarperOne, 2008.